GLYCEMIC INDEX DIET COOKBOOK FOR LOW GI

Glycemic Foods List With Delicious Healthy Snacks, Recipes, Meal Plans, the Glycemic Guidebook to GL and GI Values

Copyright © 2023.

All rights reserved. This publication and its contents are protected by copyright law. No part of this publication may be reproduced, distributed, or transmitted in any form or by any means, including photocopying, recording, or other electronic or mechanical methods, without the prior written permission of the copyright holder, except in the case of brief quotations embodied in critical reviews and other noncommercial uses permitted by copyright law. Unauthorized reproduction or distribution of this publication, in whole or in part, is strictly prohibited.

OF CONTENTS

INTRODUCTION

Steve had always been a bit on the heavier side. It wasn't something that bothered him, but he was well aware of it and was constantly trying to find ways to become healthier. He felt like he had hit a wall with his diet and exercise routine and was looking for something that could give him a little push in the right direction.

That's when he came across the Low Glycemic Index Cookbook. It was touted as a way to help people lose weight and manage their blood sugar levels. He was intrigued and decided to give it a try.

He started out by committing to a strict diet that included a lot of fresh vegetables, lean proteins, and complex carbohydrates. He cut out all added sugars and processed foods and made sure he was drinking plenty of water. He also incorporated some physical activity into his daily routine, such as walking or jogging.

At first, the changes felt overwhelming. He was used to eating whatever he wanted and not having to think too much about it. But, as the weeks went by, he started to feel better and more energized. He was losing weight, but more importantly, his blood sugar levels were improving.

Over the next few months, Steve continued to follow the diet and exercise regimen outlined in the book and was amazed at the results. He had lost a significant amount of weight and was maintaining healthy blood sugar levels. He was also feeling more energetic and capable of doing the things he wanted to do.

Steve was thrilled with the results and continued to follow the plan for the next few years. He was able to maintain his weight and blood sugar levels and had a newfound appreciation for healthy eating and physical activity. He was also able to share his success story with others, inspiring them to make healthier choices in their lives.

The Low Glycemic Index Cookbook had changed Steve's life in more ways than he could have imagined. He was now living a healthier and more fulfilling life thanks to the tips and recipes in the book.

Steve was grateful for the Low Glycemic Index Cookbook and the changes it had brought to his life. He could now enjoy the foods he loved while still staying healthy and keeping his blood sugar levels in check.

It was an incredible journey, but one that Steve was more than happy he made.

Welcome to the world of **low glycemic index cooking!** With this cookbook, you will be able to create delicious and nutritious meals that are low in sugar and high in flavor. Eating with a low glycemic index means that the food you eat will not cause a rapid spike in your blood sugar levels, which can lead to health problems such as diabetes and heart disease. Instead, you will enjoy meals that provide you with the sustenance you need without any of the risks associated with a high-sugar diet. So get ready to indulge in a variety of dishes that are both tasty and healthy!

In this cookbook, you will find recipes for breakfast, lunch, dinner, and snacks. Each recipe is designed to help you stick to a low glycemic index diet while still enjoying all of your favorite meals. All of the recipes are easy to make and require minimal ingredients, so you won't have to spend hours in the kitchen. You can also easily adjust the recipes to suit your own tastes and dietary needs. So, let's get cooking and start enjoying meals that won't leave you feeling guilty!

Let's get started!

CHAPTER 1

The Glycemic Index (GI) is a scale that measures how quickly a food raises a person's blood sugar level. Foods that are high on the GI scale cause a rapid spike in blood sugar, while foods that are low on the GI scale cause a slower, more gradual rise in blood sugar. Eating foods with a low GI can help people manage their blood sugar levels, and can be beneficial for people with diabetes or prediabetes. The GI is also used to evaluate the health benefits of different types of carbohydrates. Foods that are high on the GI scale, such as white bread, refined grains, and sugary snacks, are usually not considered healthy choices, while foods that are low on the GI scale, such as fruits, vegetables, and whole grains, are generally considered healthier choices.

The GI scale ranges from 0 to 100, with higher numbers indicating a faster rise in blood sugar levels. Foods that have a GI of 70 or higher are considered to be high on the scale, and foods that have a GI of 55 or lower are considered to be low on the scale. Foods that are moderate on the scale have a GI between 56 and 69. Low GI foods are digested more slowly, which helps to keep blood sugar levels stable. High GI foods, on the other hand, cause a rapid spike in blood sugar levels, which can lead to a crash in energy levels.

The Glycemic Index is a useful tool for people with diabetes, as well as those who are trying to maintain a healthy weight. Eating foods with a low GI can help to regulate blood sugar levels, and can help to keep hunger at bay. The GI is also useful for comparing different types of carbohydrates, as it can help to determine which foods are healthier choices.

Overall, the Glycemic Index is a useful tool for understanding how different foods affect blood sugar levels. Eating foods with a low GI can help to regulate blood sugar levels, and can help to keep hunger at bay. It can also help to compare different types of carbohydrates, and can help to determine which foods are healthier choices.

The glycemic index is an important tool for people with diabetes, as it helps them to make smart food choices that can help to manage their diabetes. Foods with a low glycemic index are digested more slowly, which helps to keep blood sugar levels more consistent and helps to avoid spikes in blood sugar. High glycemic index foods, on the other hand, can cause blood sugar levels to spike quickly, which can be dangerous for people with diabetes. The glycemic index can also be helpful for people who are trying to lose weight. Foods with a low glycemic index are often more filling and can help to reduce cravings and boost satiety. Eating a diet that is low in the glycemic index can also help to stabilize energy levels and can help to reduce sugar cravings. In addition to helping to regulate blood sugar levels and aiding in weight loss, the glycemic index can also be beneficial for people who are trying to improve their overall health. Eating a diet that is low in the glycemic index can help to reduce inflammation and can help to improve cholesterol levels. Eating a diet that is low in the glycemic index can also help to reduce the risk of certain chronic diseases, such as type 2 diabetes and heart disease.

Overall, the glycemic index is an important tool for people with diabetes, people trying to lose weight, and people trying to improve their overall health. By making smart food choices based on the glycemic index, people can make great strides towards better health.

CHAPTER 2

UNDERSTANDING LOW GLYCEMIC INDEX

The glycemic index (GI) is a tool used to measure how quickly carbohydrates are digested and absorbed into the bloodstream. Foods with a low GI (55 or lower) are digested more slowly and generally cause a slower rise in blood sugar levels than those with a high GI (70 or higher). Low GI foods can help control blood sugar levels and may also help with weight management. Low GI foods also tend to be higher in fiber and other nutrients, making them a healthier choice overall.

Low GI foods include whole grains, legumes, fruits, vegetables, and dairy products. Whole grains, such as oats, quinoa, and barley, are high in fiber and can help to keep you feeling full for longer. Legumes, such as beans, lentils, and chickpeas, are high in protein and fiber and can help regulate blood sugar levels. Fruits and vegetables are rich in vitamins, minerals, and antioxidants, and can provide important nutrients to the body. Dairy products, such as yogurt and cheese, can help to provide protein and calcium.

Low GI foods are generally healthier and can help regulate blood sugar levels and control hunger. They can also provide important nutrients and help with weight management. When choosing carbohydrates, it is generally

recommended to opt for low GI options over high GI options. Eating a balanced diet that includes a variety of low GI foods can help to ensure that you get the nutrients that you need while controlling your blood sugar levels.

In summary, understanding the glycemic index and the role that low GI foods can play in managing blood sugar levels and weight can be beneficial. Low GI foods can provide important nutrients and help to keep you feeling full for longer periods of time, making them a healthier choice overall.

BENEFITS OF LOW GLYCEMIC INDEX FOODS

Low glycemic index (GI) foods are foods that release sugars slowly into the bloodstream, helping to avoid spikes in blood sugar levels. Low GI foods have many health benefits, and they can be incorporated into a healthy diet.

Low GI foods can help regulate blood sugar levels, which is especially important for people with diabetes. These foods can also help you feel fuller for longer, making it easier to maintain a healthy weight. Low GI foods can also reduce the risk of heart disease, stroke, and other chronic diseases.

Low GI foods can also help reduce cholesterol levels and lower the risk of certain cancers. They are also a great source of dietary fiber, which can help improve digestive health. Fiber can also help reduce the risk of constipation, diverticulitis, and other digestive issues.

Low GI foods are also beneficial for people with food intolerances, as they are less likely to cause an allergic reaction. Low GI foods also contain a variety of vitamins and minerals, which can help boost the immune system and provide essential nutrients.

In conclusion, there are many benefits to consuming low GI foods. They can help regulate blood sugar levels, promote weight loss, reduce the risk of heart disease, and more. Low GI foods are also a great source of dietary fiber and vitamins and minerals. They can help improve digestive health and reduce the risk of food intolerances. For these reasons, low GI foods are an important part of a healthy diet.

Foods with a low glycemic index are those that are digested and absorbed slowly, releasing glucose into the bloodstream at a slower rate. This can help to keep blood sugar levels in check, making them an excellent choice for people with diabetes, as well as those looking to lose weight. Examples of foods with a low glycemic index include:

- Whole grains such as oats, barley, and quinoa
- Beans and legumes such as lentils, black beans, and chickpeas
- Fruits and vegetables such as apples, oranges, spinach, and broccoli
- Nuts and seeds such as almonds, walnuts, and flaxseeds
- Dairy products such as yogurt and kefir
- Fish and seafood such as salmon, tuna, and shrimp
- Lean meats such as chicken, turkey, and lean beef
- Eggs
- Olive oil
- Dark chocolate

- Vinegar-based dressings and sauces

CHAPTER 4

HOW TO FOLLOW A LOW GLYCEMIC INDEX DIET

HOW TO FOLLOW A LOW GLYCEMIC INDEX DIET

A low glycemic index diet is an eating plan that focuses on maintaining a healthy blood sugar level by choosing foods that have a low glycemic index (GI). This type of diet is often recommended for people with diabetes, as well as those looking to lose weight and improve their overall health. The goal of a low GI diet is to consume foods that have a low GI rating, which means that they cause a slower, steadier rise in blood sugar levels.

Here are some tips for following a low glycemic index diet:

- Eat a balanced diet: It is important to focus on eating a wide variety of foods from all of the food groups, including fruits, vegetables, whole grains, lean sources of protein, and healthy fats.
- Choose low GI foods: When selecting foods, focus on those with a low glycemic index rating. Examples of low GI foods include most fruits and vegetables, legumes, nuts and seeds, and dairy products.

- Limit refined carbohydrates: Refined carbohydrates, such as white bread and white pasta, have a high GI rating and can cause a rapid spike in blood sugar levels. Therefore, it is important to limit these types of foods and opt for whole grain varieties instead.

- Avoid processed foods: Processed foods are often high in sugar and refined carbohydrates, so they should be avoided. Look for foods that are minimally processed and contain little to no added sugar.

- Monitor your blood sugar: If you have diabetes, it is important to monitor your blood sugar levels regularly. This will help you determine if you are eating the right types of foods and how they affect your blood sugar levels.

Following a low glycemic index diet can help you manage your blood sugar levels and improve your overall health. By focusing on eating a balanced diet and choosing low GI foods, you can ensure that you are getting the nutrients your body needs while avoiding the potential harm of high GI foods.

Monitoring your blood sugar levels can also be helpful in determining if your diet is working for you.

CHAPTER 5

LOW GLYCEMIC INDEX MEAL PLANNING

Low glycemic index meal planning is a great way to maintain a healthy diet and help control blood sugar levels. The glycemic index is a measure of how a food affects your blood sugar levels. Foods are rated on a scale of 0 to 100, with 100 being the highest. Foods with a low glycemic index rating, such as vegetables and whole grains, cause a slower rise in blood sugar levels, while foods with a higher rating, such as white bread, potatoes and sweets, cause a faster rise in blood sugar levels.

When planning meals, choose more low glycemic index foods and fewer high glycemic index foods. Low glycemic index foods include whole grains, legumes, fruits, vegetables, nuts and seeds, and non-starchy vegetables. High glycemic index foods include white bread, white rice, potatoes, and other refined grain products.

When planning meals, try to include a balance of low and high glycemic index foods. For breakfast, try whole grain toast with a nut butter or egg and vegetable scramble. For lunch, include a salad with grilled chicken, or a wrap with hummus and vegetables. For dinner, try roasted vegetables and fish, or a bean and vegetable soup. Snacks can include a piece of fruit, a few nuts, or a handful of whole grain crackers.

Low glycemic index meal planning can help you maintain healthy blood sugar levels and achieve your health goals. Be sure to talk to your doctor or nutritionist about any dietary changes you want to make.

CHAPTER 6

DAY 1:

Breakfast: Overnight oats with chia seeds, walnuts, and

Lunch: Mediterranean salad with spinach, feta cheese, tomatoes, and olives. raspberries.

Dinner: Chicken stir fry with bell peppers, carrots, and onions

DAY 2

Breakfast: Greek yogurt with berries, almonds, and honey.

Lunch: Turkey and avocado sandwich with whole wheat bread.

Dinner: Salmon with roasted Brussels sprouts and quinoa.

DAY 3:

Breakfast: Smoothie bowl with banana, peanut butter, and almond milk.

Lunch: Lentil and quinoa salad with roasted vegetables.

Dinner: Baked salmon with asparagus and brown rice.

DAY 4

Breakfast: Omelette with mushrooms and spinach.

Lunch: Hummus and veggie wrap with whole wheat tortillas.

Dinner: Chicken and vegetable stir fry with brown rice.

DAY 5

Breakfast: Avocado toast with poached eggs.

Lunch: Salmon and quinoa bowl with roasted vegetables.

Dinner: Grilled chicken with roasted sweet potatoes and

DAY 6

Breakfast: Oatmeal with blueberries, walnuts, and honey.

Lunch: Turkey and spinach wrap with whole wheat tortillas.

Dinner: Baked cod with roasted Brussels sprouts and quinoa.

DAY 7

Breakfast: Scrambled eggs with bell peppers and onions.

Lunch: Greek salad with tomatoes, feta cheese, and olives.

Dinner: Grilled salmon with roasted sweet potatoes and asparagus.

Chapter 7

OVERNIGHT OATS WITH BERRIES AND ALMONDS – 10 MINUTES

INGREDIENTS:

- 1/2 cup rolled oats
- 1/2 cup almond milk
- 1/2 teaspoon vanilla extract
- 1 tablespoon honey
- 1/4 teaspoon ground cinnamon
- 1/2 cup fresh berries
- 2 tablespoons chopped almonds

INSTRUCTIONS:

1. In a medium bowl, combine oats, almond milk, vanilla, honey and cinnamon. Stir until evenly combined.
2. Cover bowl with plastic wrap and refrigerate overnight.
3. The next morning, remove bowl from refrigerator and stir in fresh berries and almonds.

4. Serve chilled and enjoy.

GREEK YOGURT WITH GRANOLA AND FRUIT – 5 MINUTES

INGREDIENTS:

- 1 cup plain Greek yogurt
- 1/4 cup granola
- 1/2 cup fresh berries or chopped fruit

INSTRUCTIONS:

1. In a medium bowl, combine Greek yogurt and granola.
2. Top with fresh berries or chopped fruit and enjoy.

EGG WHITE OMELET WITH SPINACH AND TOMATOES – 10 MINUTES

INGREDIENTS:

- 2 egg whites
- 1 tablespoon grated Parmesan cheese
- 1/4 teaspoon garlic powder
- 1/2 cup chopped fresh spinach
- 1/4 cup chopped tomatoes
- Salt and pepper to taste

INSTRUCTIONS:

1. In a medium bowl, whisk together egg whites, Parmesan cheese, and garlic powder until combined.
2. Heat a large non-stick skillet over medium heat.
3. Add egg mixture to skillet and cook until eggs begin to set, about 2 minutes.
4. Add spinach and tomatoes, season with salt and pepper, and cook for an additional 2 minutes.
5. Gently fold omelet in half and cook for an additional 1 minute.
6. Transfer to a plate and enjoy.

PROTEIN PANCAKES – 10 MINUTES

INGREDIENTS:

- 1/2 cup rolled oats
- 2 egg whites
- 1/4 cup plain Greek yogurt
- 1 tablespoon honey
- 1/4 teaspoon baking powder

INSTRUCTIONS:

1. In a blender, combine oats, egg whites, Greek yogurt, honey, and baking powder.
2. Blend until mixture is smooth and creamy.
3. Heat a large non-stick skillet over medium heat.
4. Add batter to skillet in 1/4 cup portions.
5. Cook pancakes for 2-3 minutes per side or until golden brown.
6. Serve with your favorite toppings and enjoy.

AVOCADO TOAST WITH EGG – 5 MINUTES

INGREDIENTS:

- 2 slices whole wheat bread
- 1/2 avocado
- 2 eggs
- Salt and pepper to taste

INSTRUCTIONS:

1. Toast bread slices.
2. Meanwhile, heat a non-stick skillet over medium-low heat.
3. Add eggs to skillet and cook for 3-4 minutes or until cooked to desired doneness.
4. Spread avocado onto toasted bread slices.
5. Top with cooked eggs, season with salt and pepper, and enjoy.

BERRY BANANA SMOOTHIE BOWL – 5 MINUTES

INGREDIENTS:

- 1/2 cup frozen berries
- 1/2 banana
- 1/4 cup plain Greek yogurt
- 1/4 cup almond milk
- 1 tablespoon honey
- 1/4 teaspoon ground cinnamon
- Toppings of your choice (granola, nuts, chia seeds, etc.)

INSTRUCTIONS:

1. In a blender, combine frozen berries, banana, Greek yogurt, almond milk, honey, and cinnamon.
2. Blend until smooth and creamy.
3. Pour smoothie into a bowl and top with desired toppings.
4. Serve and enjoy.

QUINOA BREAKFAST BOWL – 10 MINUTES

INGREDIENTS:

- 1/2 cup cooked quinoa

* 1/4 cup chopped almonds
* 1/4 cup chopped fresh fruit
* 1/4 cup plain Greek yogurt
* 1 tablespoon honey

INSTRUCTIONS:

1. In a medium bowl, combine cooked quinoa, almonds, fruit, Greek yogurt, and honey.
2. Stir until evenly combined.
3. Serve and enjoy.

SAVORY OATMEAL WITH SPINACH AND FETA – 10 MINUTES

INGREDIENTS:

* 1/2 cup rolled oats
* 1/2 cup vegetable broth
* 1/4 cup chopped fresh spinach
* 1 tablespoon crumbled feta cheese
* Salt and pepper to taste

INSTRUCTIONS:

1. In a medium saucepan, bring vegetable broth to a boil.

2. Add oats and cook for 5 minutes, stirring occasionally.
3. Stir in spinach and cook for an additional 2 minutes.
4. Remove from heat and stir in feta cheese. Season with salt and pepper to taste.
5. Serve and enjoy.

SWEET POTATO TOAST – 5 MINUTES

INGREDIENTS:

- 2 slices sweet potato
- 1 tablespoon peanut butter
- 1/4 cup sliced banana

INSTRUCTIONS:

1. Toast sweet potato slices in a toaster or toaster oven.
2. Spread peanut butter on toasted sweet potato slices.
3. Top with sliced banana and enjoy.

WHOLE WHEAT BLUEBERRY MUFFINS – 10 MINUTES

INGREDIENTS:

- 1 cup whole wheat flour
- 1/2 teaspoon baking powder
- 1/2 teaspoon baking soda
- 1/4 teaspoon ground cinnamon
- 1/4 cup honey
- 1/4 cup almond milk
- 1/4 cup melted coconut oil
- 1 egg
- 1/2 cup fresh blueberries

INSTRUCTIONS:

1. Preheat oven to 375°F.
2. In a medium bowl, whisk together flour, baking powder, baking soda, and cinnamon.
3. In a separate bowl, whisk together honey, almond milk, coconut oil, and egg.
4. Pour wet ingredients into dry and stir until just combined.
5. Gently fold in blueberries.
6. Divide batter evenly among prepared muffin tins.
7. Bake for 15-20 minutes or until a toothpick inserted into center comes out clean.
8. Allow to cool before serving. Enjoy.

MEDITERRANEAN CHICKEN WRAP: PREP TIME: 10 MINS

INGREDIENTS:

- 4 whole-wheat wraps
- 4 tablespoons hummus
- 4 ounces roasted chicken breast, sliced
- 1/4 cup sliced cucumber
- 1/4 cup sliced red bell pepper
- 1/4 cup sliced Kalamata olives
- 1/4 cup feta cheese

INSTRUCTIONS:

1. Spread 1 tablespoon of hummus onto each wrap.
2. Divide chicken, cucumber, bell pepper, olives and feta among the wraps.
3. Roll up the wraps and enjoy!

QUINOA AND SPINACH SALAD: PREP TIME: 10 MINS

INGREDIENTS:

- 1 cup cooked quinoa
- 2 cups baby spinach
- 1/2 cup cooked black beans
- 1/2 cup diced tomatoes
- 1/4 cup diced red onion
- 1/4 cup diced cucumber
- 2 tablespoons olive oil
- 2 tablespoons balsamic vinegar
- Salt and pepper to taste

INSTRUCTIONS:

1. In a medium bowl, combine quinoa, spinach, black beans, tomatoes, red onion and cucumber.
2. In a small bowl, whisk together olive oil, balsamic vinegar, salt and pepper.

3. Pour dressing over the quinoa and vegetable mixture and toss to combine.
4. Serve chilled or at room temperature.

LENTIL AND AVOCADO WRAP: PREP TIME: 10 MINS

INGREDIENTS:

- 4 whole-wheat wraps
- 1 cup cooked lentils
- 2 avocados, mashed
- 1/4 cup diced red onion
- 1/4 cup diced bell peppers
- 1/4 cup crumbled feta cheese
- Salt and pepper to taste

INSTRUCTIONS:

1. Spread 1/4 of the mashed avocado onto each wrap.
2. Divide lentils, onion, bell peppers and feta among the wraps.
3. Sprinkle with salt and pepper to taste.

4. Roll up the wraps and enjoy!

EGG AND VEGGIE SANDWICH: PREP TIME: 10 MINS

INGREDIENTS:

- 4 whole-wheat English muffins
- 4 eggs, cooked
- 1/4 cup sliced mushrooms
- 1/4 cup diced bell peppers
- 1/4 cup diced red onion
- 2 tablespoons olive oil
- Salt and pepper to taste

INSTRUCTIONS:

1. Split the English muffins and spread 1/2 tablespoon of olive oil on each side.
2. Divide eggs, mushrooms, bell peppers, and red onion among the English muffins.
3. Sprinkle with salt and pepper to taste.

4. Top with remaining English muffin halves and enjoy!

TURKEY AND VEGGIE WRAP: PREP TIME: 10 MINS

INGREDIENTS:

- 4 whole-wheat wraps
- 4 ounces roasted turkey breast, sliced
- 1/4 cup diced bell peppers
- 1/4 cup diced cucumber
- 1/4 cup crumbled feta cheese
- 2 tablespoons olive oil
- Salt and pepper to taste

INSTRUCTIONS:

1. Spread 1/2 tablespoon of olive oil onto each wrap.
2. Divide turkey, bell peppers, cucumber and feta among the wraps.
3. Sprinkle with salt and pepper to taste.

4. Roll up the wraps and enjoy!

CHICKPEA AND TOMATO SALAD: PREP TIME: 10 MINS

INGREDIENTS:

- 1 can chickpeas, drained and rinsed
- 1 cup diced tomatoes
- 1/4 cup diced red onion
- 1/4 cup diced cucumber
- 2 tablespoons olive oil
- 2 tablespoons balsamic vinegar
- Salt and pepper to taste

INSTRUCTIONS:

1. In a medium bowl, combine chickpeas, tomatoes, red onion and cucumber.
2. In a small bowl, whisk together olive oil, balsamic vinegar, salt and pepper.

3. Pour dressing over the chickpea and vegetable mixture and toss to combine.
4. Serve chilled or at room temperature.

BEET AND AVOCADO SALAD: PREP TIME: 10 MINS

INGREDIENTS:

- 2 cups baby spinach
- 1/2 cup cooked beets, diced
- 1/4 cup diced red onion
- 1/4 cup diced bell peppers
- 2 tablespoons olive oil
- 2 tablespoons balsamic vinegar
- 1 avocado, diced
- Salt and pepper to taste

INSTRUCTIONS:

1. In a medium bowl, combine spinach, beets, onion and bell peppers.
2. In a small bowl, whisk together olive oil, balsamic vinegar, salt and pepper.

3. Pour dressing over the spinach and vegetable mixture and toss to combine.
4. Top with diced avocado.
5. Serve chilled or at room temperature.

TURKEY AND CHEESE SANDWICH: PREP TIME: 10 MINS

INGREDIENTS:

- 4 whole-wheat slices of bread
- 4 ounces roasted turkey breast, sliced
- 4 slices low-fat cheese
- 1/4 cup diced tomatoes
- 1/4 cup diced red onion
- 2 tablespoons olive oil
- Salt and pepper to taste

INSTRUCTIONS:

1. Spread 1/2 tablespoon of olive oil onto each slice of bread.
2. Divide turkey, cheese, tomatoes and red onion among the slices of bread.

3. Sprinkle with salt and pepper to taste.
4. Top with remaining slices of bread and enjoy!

CUCUMBER AND HUMMUS WRAP: PREP TIME: 10 MINS

INGREDIENTS:

- 4 whole-wheat wraps
- 4 tablespoons hummus
- 1/2 cup sliced cucumber
- 1/4 cup diced bell peppers
- 1/4 cup crumbled feta cheese
- 2 tablespoons olive oil
- Salt and pepper to taste

INSTRUCTIONS:

1. Spread 1 tablespoon of hummus onto each wrap.
2. Divide cucumber, bell peppers and feta among the wraps.

3. Drizzle with olive oil and sprinkle with salt and pepper to taste.
4. Roll up the wraps and enjoy!

GREEK YOGURT AND FRUIT BOWL: PREP TIME: 10 MINS

INGREDIENTS:

- 4 cups Greek yogurt
- 1/2 cup diced strawberries
- 1/2 cup diced blueberries
- 1/4 cup diced mango
- 1/4 cup diced kiwi
- 2 tablespoons honey

INSTRUCTIONS:

1. In a medium bowl, combine yogurt, strawberries, blueberries, mango and kiwi.
2. Drizzle with honey and stir to combine.
3. Serve chilled or at room temperature.

SOUTHWESTERN STUFFED PEPPERS – PREP TIME: 15 MINUTES

INGREDIENTS:

- 4 bell peppers, halved lengthwise, seeds and membranes removed
- 1 tablespoon olive oil
- 1 onion, diced
- 1 garlic clove, minced
- 1 teaspoon ground cumin
- 1/2 teaspoon chili powder
- 1/2 teaspoon dried oregano
- 1/2 teaspoon paprika
- 1/2 teaspoon salt
- 1/4 teaspoon black pepper
- 1 1/2 cups cooked quinoa
- 1 can black beans, rinsed and drained
- 1/2 cup frozen corn
- 1/2 cup salsa
- 1/2 cup shredded Monterey Jack cheese

INSTRUCTIONS:

1. Preheat oven to 375 degrees F.
2. Place pepper halves in a large baking dish.
3. Heat olive oil in a large skillet over medium heat. Add onion and garlic and cook until softened, about 5 minutes.
4. Add cumin, chili powder, oregano, paprika, salt, and black pepper and cook until fragrant, about 1 minute.
5. Stir in quinoa, beans, corn, and salsa. Cook until heated through, about 5 minutes.
6. Stuff the pepper halves with the quinoa mixture and top with cheese.
7. Bake in preheated oven for 20 minutes, or until the peppers are tender.

BAKED SALMON WITH COCONUT LIME SAUCE – PREP TIME: 15 MINUTES

INGREDIENTS:

- 1/2 cup canned coconut milk
- 2 tablespoons fresh lime juice

- 1/2 teaspoon grated lime zest
- 1/4 teaspoon sea salt
- 4 (4-ounce) skinless salmon fillets
- 1 tablespoon olive oil
- 1 tablespoon finely chopped fresh cilantro

INSTRUCTIONS:

1. Preheat oven to 400 degrees F.
2. In a small bowl, whisk together coconut milk, lime juice, lime zest, and salt.
3. Place salmon fillets in a greased baking dish and brush with olive oil.
4. Pour the coconut milk mixture over the salmon.
5. Bake in preheated oven for 12–15 minutes, or until fish is cooked through.
6. Sprinkle with cilantro before serving.

ZUCCHINI NOODLES WITH AVOCADO PESTO – PREP TIME: 10 MINUTES

INGREDIENTS:

- 2 large zucchinis, spiralized
- 1/2 cup fresh basil leaves
- 1/4 cup olive oil

- 1 avocado, diced
- 2 cloves garlic, minced
- 1/4 teaspoon sea salt
- 1/4 teaspoon black pepper
- 1/4 cup freshly grated Parmesan cheese

INSTRUCTIONS:

1. Place zucchini noodles in a large bowl.
2. In a food processor, combine basil, olive oil, avocado, garlic, salt, and pepper and pulse until smooth.
3. Pour the pesto over the noodles and toss to combine.
4. Sprinkle with Parmesan cheese before serving.

VEGETARIAN CHILI – PREP TIME: 10 MINUTES

INGREDIENTS:

- 1 tablespoon olive oil
- 1 onion, diced

- 2 cloves garlic, minced
- 2 teaspoons ground cumin
- 1 teaspoon chili powder
- 1/2 teaspoon dried oregano
- 1/2 teaspoon paprika
- 1/4 teaspoon cayenne pepper
- 1 can black beans, rinsed and drained
- 1 can diced tomatoes
- 1 can corn, drained
- 1/4 cup vegetable broth

INSTRUCTIONS:

1. Heat olive oil in a large pot over medium heat.
2. Add onion and garlic and cook until softened, about 5 minutes.
3. Add cumin, chili powder, oregano, paprika, and cayenne pepper and cook until fragrant, about 1 minute.
4. Stir in black beans, tomatoes, corn, and broth.
5. Bring to a boil, reduce heat, and simmer for 10 minutes.

EGGPLANT AND LENTIL CURRY – PREP TIME: 10 MINUTES

INGREDIENTS:

- 1 tablespoon olive oil
- 1 onion, diced
- 2 cloves garlic, minced
- 1 teaspoon ground cumin
- 1 teaspoon ground coriander
- 1/2 teaspoon ground turmeric
- 1/2 teaspoon ground ginger
- 1/4 teaspoon cayenne pepper
- 1 eggplant, diced
- 1 can lentils, rinsed and drained
- 1 can diced tomatoes
- 1/4 cup vegetable broth

INSTRUCTIONS:

1. Heat olive oil in a large pot over medium heat.
2. Add onion and garlic and cook until softened, about 5 minutes.

3. Add cumin, coriander, turmeric, ginger, and cayenne pepper and cook until fragrant, about 1 minute.
4. Stir in eggplant, lentils, tomatoes, and broth.
5. Bring to a boil, reduce heat, and simmer for 10 minutes.

MEDITERRANEAN QUINOA SALAD – PREP TIME: 15 MINUTES

INGREDIENTS:

- 1 cup quinoa, cooked
- 1 cucumber, diced
- 1 tomato, diced
- 1/2 cup kalamata olives, sliced
- 1/4 cup feta cheese, crumbled
- 1/4 cup olive oil
- 2 tablespoons red wine vinegar
- 1 teaspoon dried oregano
- 1/2 teaspoon garlic powder
- 1/4 teaspoon sea salt

INSTRUCTIONS:

1. In a large bowl, combine quinoa, cucumber, tomato, olives, and feta cheese.

2. In a small bowl, whisk together olive oil, red wine vinegar, oregano, garlic powder, and salt.
3. Pour dressing over quinoa mixture and toss to combine.

ROASTED SWEET POTATO SALAD – PREP TIME: 20 MINUTES

INGREDIENTS:

- 2 large sweet potatoes, peeled and diced
- 2 tablespoons olive oil
- 1/2 teaspoon sea salt
- 1/4 teaspoon black pepper
- 1/4 teaspoon garlic powder
- 1/4 cup chopped fresh parsley
- 1/4 cup chopped fresh mint
- 1/4 cup diced red onion
- 1/4 cup feta cheese, crumbled
- 1/4 cup toasted sliced almonds

INSTRUCTIONS:

1. Preheat oven to 375 degrees F.
2. Place sweet potatoes on a baking sheet and drizzle with olive oil.

3. Sprinkle with salt, pepper, and garlic powder.

4. Roast in preheated oven for 20 minutes, or until tender.

5. In a large bowl, combine parsley, mint, red onion, feta cheese, and almonds.

6. Add roasted sweet potatoes and toss to combine.

LENTIL AND KALE SOUP – PREP TIME: 10 MINUTES

INGREDIENTS:

- 1 tablespoon olive oil
- 1 onion, diced
- 2 cloves garlic, minced
- 1 teaspoon ground cumin
- 1/2 teaspoon dried oregano
- 1/4 teaspoon cayenne pepper
- 1 can diced tomatoes
- 1 can lentils, rinsed and drained
- 4 cups vegetable broth
- 2 cups chopped kale

INSTRUCTIONS:

1. Heat olive oil in a large pot over medium heat.
2. Add onion and garlic and cook until softened, about 5 minutes.
3. Add cumin, oregano, and cayenne pepper and cook until fragrant, about 1 minute.
4. Stir in tomatoes, lentils, and broth.
5. Bring to a boil, reduce heat, and simmer for 10 minutes.
6. Stir in kale and cook until wilted, about 5 minutes.

CAULIFLOWER RICE BURRITO BOWLS – PREP TIME: 10 MINUTES

INGREDIENTS:

*   1 tablespoon olive oil

- 1 onion, diced
- 1 bell pepper, diced
- 1 garlic clove, minced
- 1 teaspoon ground cumin
- 1/2 teaspoon chili powder
- 1/2 teaspoon dried oregano
- 1/2 teaspoon paprika
- 1/4 teaspoon sea salt
- 1/4 teaspoon black pepper
- 1 head cauliflower, grated
- 1 can black beans, rinsed and drained
- 1 can corn, drained
- 1/2 cup salsa

INSTRUCTIONS:

1. Heat olive oil in a large skillet over medium heat.
2. Add onion, bell pepper, and garlic and cook until softened, about 5 minutes.
3. Add cumin, chili powder, oregano, paprika, salt, and black pepper and cook until fragrant, about 1 minute.
4. Stir in cauliflower, beans, and corn and cook until heated through, about 5 minutes.
5. Serve in bowls with salsa.

SLOW COOKER VEGGIE LASAGNA – PREP TIME: 10 MINUTES

INGREDIENTS:

- 1 onion, diced
- 2 cloves garlic, minced
- 1 can diced tomatoes
- 1 can tomato sauce
- 1 teaspoon dried oregano
- 1/2 teaspoon dried basil
- 1/2 teaspoon sea salt
- 1/4 teaspoon black pepper
- 2 cups spinach
- 1/2 cup ricotta cheese
- 1/2 cup shredded mozzarella cheese
- 1/4 cup freshly grated Parmesan cheese

INSTRUCTIONS:

1. Place onion and garlic in the bottom of a slow cooker.
2. Add diced tomatoes, tomato sauce, oregano, basil, salt, and pepper and stir to combine.

3. Top with spinach, ricotta cheese, and mozzarella cheese.
4. Cover and cook on low for 4–6 hours.
5. Sprinkle with Parmesan cheese before serving.

Low Glycemic Index Snack Recipes

BANANA OAT BITES

PREP TIME: 10 MINUTES

INGREDIENTS:

- 2 ripe bananas
- 2 cups rolled oats
- 2 tablespoons melted coconut oil
- 2 tablespoons honey

INSTRUCTIONS:

1. Preheat oven to 350°F.
2. Mash bananas in a medium bowl until smooth.
3. Stir in oats, coconut oil, and honey until combined.
4. Drop spoonfuls of the mixture onto a baking sheet lined with parchment paper.
5. Bake for 12-15 minutes until golden brown.
6. Allow to cool before serving.

PEANUT BUTTER APPLE BITES

PREP TIME: 10 MINUTES

INGREDIENTS:

- 2 apples, cored and sliced
- 2 tablespoons peanut butter
- 2 tablespoons honey

INSTRUCTIONS:

1. Spread peanut butter over each apple slice.
2. Drizzle honey over the peanut butter.
3. Enjoy!

TRAIL MIX

PREP TIME: 10 MINUTES

INGREDIENTS:

- 1/2 cup almonds
- 1/2 cup walnuts
- 1/2 cup dried cranberries
- 1/2 cup dried banana chips

INSTRUCTIONS:

1. Combine almonds, walnuts, cranberries, and banana chips in a bowl.
2. Mix until ingredients are evenly distributed.
3. Enjoy!

VEGGIE HUMMUS WRAP

PREP TIME: 10 MINUTES

INGREDIENTS:

- 1 whole wheat tortilla
- 2 tablespoons hummus
- 1/4 cup spinach
- 1/4 cup shredded carrots
- 1/4 cup diced peppers

INSTRUCTIONS:

1. Spread hummus onto the tortilla.
2. Top with spinach, carrots, and peppers.
3. Roll up and enjoy!

GREEK YOGURT PARFAIT

PREP TIME: 10 MINUTES

INGREDIENTS:

- 1/2 cup Greek yogurt
- 1/4 cup granola
- 1/4 cup fresh berries

INSTRUCTIONS:

1. Layer yogurt, granola, and berries into a bowl.
2. Enjoy!

APPLE WALNUT SALAD

PREP TIME: 10 MINUTES

INGREDIENTS:

- 2 apples, diced
- 1/4 cup walnuts
- 2 tablespoons honey
- 2 tablespoons olive oil
- 2 tablespoons lemon juice

INSTRUCTIONS:

1. Combine apples, walnuts, honey, olive oil, and lemon juice in a bowl.
2. Mix until ingredients are evenly distributed.
3. Enjoy!

BAKED SWEET POTATO FRIES

PREP TIME: 10 MINUTES

INGREDIENTS:

- 2 sweet potatoes, cut into fries
- 2 tablespoons olive oil
- 1 teaspoon garlic powder
- 1 teaspoon paprika

INSTRUCTIONS:

1. Preheat oven to 425°F.
2. Toss sweet potatoes in olive oil, garlic powder, and paprika.
3. Spread fries onto a baking sheet lined with parchment paper.
4. Bake for 15-20 minutes until golden brown.
5. Enjoy!

OATMEAL ENERGY BITES

PREP TIME: 10 MINUTES

INGREDIENTS:

- 1/2 cup rolled oats
- 2 tablespoons peanut butter
- 2 tablespoons honey
- 1/4 cup dried cranberries

INSTRUCTIONS:

1. Combine oats, peanut butter, honey, and cranberries in a bowl.
2. Mix until ingredients are evenly distributed.
3. Roll into balls and enjoy!

QUINOA SALAD

PREP TIME: 10 MINUTES

INGREDIENTS:

- 1 cup cooked quinoa
- 1/2 cup black beans
- 1/2 cup diced tomatoes
- 2 tablespoons olive oil
- 2 tablespoons lime juice

INSTRUCTIONS:

1. Combine quinoa, black beans, and tomatoes in a bowl.
2. Add olive oil and lime juice and mix until ingredients are evenly distributed.
3. Enjoy!

PUMPKIN PIE SMOOTHIE

PREP TIME: 10 MINUTES

INGREDIENTS:

- 1 banana
- 1/2 cup pumpkin puree
- 1/2 cup almond milk
- 1/4 teaspoon pumpkin pie spice

INSTRUCTIONS:

1. Place banana, pumpkin puree, almond milk, and pumpkin pie spice in a blender.
2. Blend until smooth.
3. Enjoy!

Low Glycemic Index Smoothies

Recipes

BLUEBERRY BANANA SMOOTHIE: PREP TIME: 5 MINUTES,

INGREDIENTS:

- 1/2 cup frozen blueberries,
- 1 banana,
- 1 cup almond milk,
- 1 tablespoon almond butter,
- 1/4 teaspoon cinnamon,

INSTRUCTIONS:

1. Blend all ingredients together in a blender until smooth.
2. Enjoy!

This smoothie is a great way to start your day and fuel your body with plenty of healthy nutrients. The combination of blueberries, banana, almond milk, almond butter, and cinnamon makes for a delicious and nutritious smoothie with a low glycemic index. The almond milk and almond butter provide healthy fats and protein while the blueberries and banana give the smoothie a sweet and naturally sweet flavor.

The cinnamon adds a hint of spice and helps to regulate blood sugar levels.

GREEN TEA SMOOTHIE: PREP TIME: 5 MINUTES,

INGREDIENTS:

- 1 cup brewed green tea,
- 1/2 cup frozen spinach,
- 1/2 banana,
- 1/4 cup Greek yogurt,
- 1 tablespoon honey,

INSTRUCTIONS:

1. Blend all ingredients together in a blender until smooth.
2. Enjoy!

This green tea smoothie is a great way to get an energy boost and still maintain a low glycemic index. The combination of green tea, spinach, banana, Greek yogurt, and honey provides a great balance of antioxidants, fiber, protein, and healthy fats that will keep your blood sugar levels steady. The green tea and spinach provide a great source of antioxidants, while the banana and Greek yogurt help to add a sweet flavor. The honey adds a touch of sweetness while also helping to regulate blood sugar levels.

MANGO COCONUT SMOOTHIE: PREP TIME: 5 MINUTES,

INGREDIENTS:

- 1/2 cup frozen mango,
- 1/2 cup coconut milk,
- 1/4 cup Greek yogurt,
- 1 tablespoon chia seeds,

INSTRUCTIONS:

1. Blend all ingredients together in a blender until smooth.
2. Enjoy!

This mango coconut smoothie is a great way to get a delicious and nutritious low glycemic index snack. The combination of mango, coconut milk, Greek yogurt, and chia seeds make for a creamy and refreshing smoothie that is packed with healthy nutrients. The mango and coconut milk provide a sweet and tropical flavor while the Greek yogurt and chia seeds help to add protein and healthy fats. The chia seeds also help to regulate blood sugar levels, making this a great snack for those who are looking to maintain a healthy diet.

OATMEAL SMOOTHIE: PREP TIME: 5 MINUTES,

INGREDIENTS:

- 1/2 cup oats,
- 1 banana,
- 1 cup almond milk,
- 1 tablespoon peanut butter,

INSTRUCTIONS:

1. Blend all ingredients together in a blender until smooth.
2. Enjoy!

This oatmeal smoothie is a great way to get a nutritious snack that is low in glycemic index. The combination of oats, banana, almond milk, and peanut butter create a creamy and delicious smoothie that will keep you fuller for longer. The oats and banana provide plenty of fiber and help to regulate blood sugar levels. The almond milk and peanut butter provide healthy fats and proteins, making this an ideal snack for anyone looking to maintain a healthy diet.

AVOCADO SMOOTHIE: PREP TIME: 5 MINUTES,

INGREDIENTS:

- 1 avocado,
- 1/2 cup almond milk,
- 1/2 cup Greek yogurt,
- 1 tablespoon honey,

INSTRUCTIONS:

1. Blend all ingredients together in a blender until smooth.
2. Enjoy!

This avocado smoothie is a great way to get a healthy and delicious snack that has a low glycemic index. The combination of avocado, almond milk, Greek yogurt, and honey provides a creamy and delicious smoothie that is packed with healthy nutrients. The avocado and almond milk provide healthy fats and proteins while the Greek yogurt and honey give the smoothie a sweet and naturally sweet flavor. The honey also helps to regulate blood sugar levels, making this a great snack for those who are looking to maintain a healthy diet.

APPLE CINNAMON SMOOTHIE: PREP TIME: 5 MINUTES,

INGREDIENTS:

- 1 apple,
- 1 banana,
- 1 cup almond milk,
- 1/4 teaspoon cinnamon,

INSTRUCTIONS:

1. Blend all ingredients together in a blender until smooth.
2. Enjoy!

This apple cinnamon smoothie is a great way to get a nutritious snack that has a low glycemic index. The combination of apple, banana, almond milk, and cinnamon creates a delicious and creamy smoothie that is packed with healthy nutrients. The apple and banana provide plenty of fiber and help to regulate blood sugar levels. The almond milk and cinnamon add a naturally sweet flavor and help to provide a boost of energy.

CHOCOLATE PEANUT BUTTER SMOOTHIE: PREP TIME: 5 MINUTES,

INGREDIENTS:

- 1 banana,
- 1/2 cup almond milk,
- 1 tablespoon cocoa powder,
- 1 tablespoon peanut butter,

INSTRUCTIONS:

1. Blend all ingredients together in a blender until smooth.
2. Enjoy!

This chocolate peanut butter smoothie is a great way to get a delicious and nutritious snack that has a low glycemic index. The combination of banana, almond milk, cocoa powder, and peanut butter creates a creamy and delicious smoothie that is packed with healthy nutrients. The banana and almond milk provide plenty of fiber and help to regulate blood sugar levels. The cocoa powder and peanut butter add a rich and naturally sweet flavor while also providing healthy fats and proteins.

STRAWBERRY BANANA SMOOTHIE: PREP TIME: 5 MINUTES,

INGREDIENTS:

- 1/2 cup frozen strawberries,
- 1 banana,
- 1 cup almond milk,
- 1 tablespoon chia seeds,

INSTRUCTIONS:

1. Blend all ingredients together in a blender until smooth.
2. Enjoy!

This strawberry banana smoothie is a great way to get a delicious and nutritious snack that has a low glycemic index. The combination of strawberries, banana, almond milk, and chia seeds create a creamy and delicious smoothie that is packed with healthy nutrients. The strawberries and banana provide plenty of fiber and help to regulate blood sugar levels. The almond milk and chia seeds add a naturally sweet flavor while also providing healthy fats and proteins.

CARROT ORANGE SMOOTHIE: PREP TIME: 5 MINUTES,

INGREDIENTS:

- 1/2 cup carrots,
- 1/2 cup orange juice,
- 1/2 cup Greek yogurt,
- 1 tablespoon honey,

INSTRUCTIONS:

1. Blend all ingredients together in a blender until smooth.
2. Enjoy!

This carrot orange smoothie is a great way to get a nutritious snack that has a low glycemic index. The combination of carrots, orange juice, Greek yogurt, and honey create a delicious and creamy smoothie that is packed with healthy nutrients. The carrots and orange juice provide plenty of fiber and help to regulate blood sugar levels. The Greek yogurt and honey add a naturally sweet flavor while also providing healthy fats and proteins.

SPINACH BANANA SMOOTHIE: PREP TIME: 5 MINUTES,

INGREDIENTS:

- 1/2 cup frozen spinach,
- 1 banana,
- 1 cup almond milk,
- 1 tablespoon chia seeds,

INSTRUCTIONS:

1. Blend all ingredients together in a blender until smooth.
2. Enjoy!

This spinach banana smoothie is a great way to get a nutritious snack that has a low glycemic index. The combination of spinach, banana, almond milk, and chia seeds make for a creamy and delicious smoothie that is packed with healthy nutrients. The spinach and banana provide plenty of fiber and help to regulate blood sugar levels. The almond milk and chia seeds add a naturally sweet flavor while also providing healthy fats and proteins.

Chapter 8

CONCLUSION

Low glycemic index foods are an essential part of any healthy diet as they have been shown to have a range of positive health benefits. Eating low glycemic index foods helps to maintain stable blood sugar levels, reducing the risk of developing type 2 diabetes and other chronic diseases. Additionally, low glycemic index foods make us feel fuller for longer and can help to reduce cravings, making them an effective tool for weight loss.

Low glycemic index foods generally consist of unprocessed, whole foods such as fruits, vegetables, whole grains, legumes, nuts, and seeds. These foods are not only low in glycemic index but are also packed with vitamins, minerals, and other essential nutrients that are necessary for a healthy body and mind. Furthermore, they are usually low in calories and fat but still provide the body with the energy and nutrition it needs to function properly.

Incorporating low glycemic index foods into your diet is a great way to boost your overall health and wellbeing. Eating these foods on a regular basis can help to improve your energy levels, reduce hunger and cravings, and even aid in weight loss. Low glycemic index foods also have many other health benefits, such as reducing the risk of developing chronic diseases, improving digestive health, and promoting heart health.

Making sure to include low glycemic index foods in your diet is a great way to ensure that you are getting the nutrition you need without increasing your risk of developing chronic diseases. Eating a variety of low glycemic index foods can help to improve your overall health and wellbeing and can make a significant difference in your day-to-day life.

In summary, low glycemic index foods are nutritious, low-calorie options that are beneficial for overall health. Eating a diet rich in low glycemic index foods can help to maintain stable blood sugar levels, reduce hunger and cravings, improve energy levels, and even aid in weight loss. Incorporating these foods into your diet is a great way to ensure that you are getting the nutrition you need without increasing your risk of developing chronic diseases.